Pocket E

GW00367888

Aromatnerapy

Kevin Hudson

Astrolog Publishing House

Pocket Healing Books

Holistic Healing
Dr. Ilona Melman

Aromatherapy
Kevin Hudson

Reiki
Chantal Dupont

Vitamins
Jon Tillman

Introduction

Aromatherapy is the art of using the essential oils extracted from plants both for healing purposes and for improving quality of life. Essential oils have been used since the dawn of mankind for healing. Some of them, such as myrrh, frankincense, hyssop, and so on, are mentioned in the Bible. They are all antiseptic, without exception, as well as fungicidal, viricidal, and anti-inflammatory. They do not have the side-effects found in synthetic medications; perhaps this accounts for the renewed interest in natural healing.

Essential oils are absorbed into the body through the skin, and reach the circulatory system, thereby affecting the entire body. Their fragrance exerts a great psychological influence: they stimulate or relax, enhance or decrease sexual desire, and so on. They are useful in treating various psychological conditions.

Because of their healing properties, essential oils are very effective in treating a wide variety of skin problems. In combination with relaxing oils, there is a combined mental-physical effect that accelerates healing.

The quality of the oils is extremely important. As it is difficult to determine, the best method is to purchase the oils only from a reliable source.

Essential oils, extracted from plants, contain volatile compounds. These oils are contained in minute amounts in the plant cells, and their function is to protect the cells from diseases and pests, as well as to attract certain insects for the purpose of pollination. Sometimes the oil serves as a natural poison secreted by the roots, in order to prevent other plants from growing too close to it.

Essential oils are produced from different parts of the plants: Flowers, leaves, roots, peel, resin, and so on. They are characterized by their strong odor and their healing properties. The quality of the oil depends on the part of the plant from which it was produced. For instance, angelica oil that is produced from the root of the plant is of much higher quality than that which comes from its seeds.

Essential oils are not water-soluble, but dissolve well in alcohol, and blend easily with macerated oils, fats, and wax.

How essential oils are extracted from plants:

By immersion in oil - the most ancient method. Plant parts are immersed in a stable oil, such as almond oil, at a relatively high temperature, for a few days to a few weeks. The plant remnants are strained off, and the oil is ready for use. The essential oil produced by this method is not absolutely pure, but rather a mixture of essential oil and macerated oil.

By squeezing - a very common method, used for extracting oil from citrus peel. The peel undergoes a process of pressing or mashing and squeezing by centrifuge.

By distillation - the most common method. This involves condensation apparatus, by means of which water is boiled, and the steam passes through a pipe and reaches a container with the plant parts, causing the oil from the plants to evaporate. A mixture of plant and water steam passes through a cooling pipe, condenses, and drips down into another container. Because of the difference in specific gravity, the water, which is heavier, sinks to the bottom, while the oil floats (except for clove and benzoin oil, which sink to the bottom.)

By enfleurage - the most delicate and expensive method. A glass slab in a wooden frame is covered with oil, upon which a layer of fresh flowers is sprinkled. A day later, all the oil in the flowers is absorbed into the oil layer, and they are replaced by a fresh layer of flowers. This procedure is repeated for over two months until the oil is saturated with essential oil. The fat which is saturated with essential oil is called "pomade." The next stage is dissolving the essential oil in alcohol by shaking the frame constantly. The fat, however, does not dissolve. Then the alcohol is evaporated, and the pure, essential oil remains.

By dissolving in a solvent - a modern method whose aim is to produce as much oil as possible within a short time. The plants are placed in a container with a solvent such as acetone, xylene, etc. The mixture is heated, and the essential oil dissolves in the solvent together with the plant's natural wax. The plant remnants are strained off, the solvent is evaporated, leaving a thick, dark paste called "concrete," which is mixed with alcohol and refrigerated. The essential oil dissolves in the alcohol, while the wax remains as a residue. The solution is strained, the alcohol is evaporated, and the essential oil remains.

How to use essential oils:

Massage - Massaging the body is soothing and relaxing; it stimulates the circulatory system, and creates an overall good feeling. Add essential oils to this, and the advantages are even greater. The proportion of vegetable oil to essential oil is 97.5:2.5%, or to every 2 ml of vegetable oil, one drop of essential oil is added.

Bath - This is also relaxing, and a good way of making the most of the essential oils, as they are not water-soluble, and they float on the surface of the water. In order to spread the oil evenly throughout the bath-water, one of the following methods can be used: (i) Place one heaped tablespoon of bath salts, epsom salts or cooking salt and 5 drops of essential oil in half a glass of lukewarm water, and add to the bath. (ii) While filling the bath, pour one tablespoon of shampoo or liquid soap and 5 drops of essential oil into the water. This method can also be used for shampooing the hair. (iii) While filling the bath, add three tablespoons of honey and 5 drops of essential oil to the water. (The honey itself is nourishing for the skin.)

Essential oil burner - The upper part of the

burner looks like a small bowl. A little water is poured into it, and 10-12 drops of essential oil added to it. (The amount of oil depends on the size of the room). The lower part of the burner contains a candle, which heats the water, causing the essential oil to evaporate and spread throughout the room. This method is very effective when someone has a contagious disease. The essential oil disinfects the air and prevents the spread of the infection. The method is also popular for creating a particular atmosphere.

Inhalation - This method is effective in cases of colds, sore throats, and so on, *but must not be used by people who suffer from asthma*. A quart of hot water is poured into a wide bowl, 5 drops of essential oil are added, the head and bowl are covered with a towel, and the steam is inhaled for a few minutes.

Precautions to be taken when using essential oils

Because essential oils are highly concentrated, certain precautions must be taken when using them.

They must never be swallowed! As they are absorbed efficiently by the skin, they are for *external use only.*

Essential oils must be stored out of the reach of children.

Essential oils must not be used undiluted on the body (unless indicated in the book). When used for a massage, they must be diluted in vegetable oil.

Before using an essential oil, it is necessary to know its properties and if its use is prohibited in any way (for instance, by pregnant women, children, etc.)

Storing essential oils

Essential oils must be stored in dark-colored, well-sealed glass (not plastic) bottles, in order to prevent the penetration of light and air. They should not be exposed to extremes of temperature, and should be stored in a cool, dark place, such as a refrigerator or a closet.

Under the correct storage conditions, most essential oils are effective for three years.

Note: The storage conditions for vegetable oils are the same as for essential oils. However, before they are mixed with essential oils, they can be stored in well-sealed plastic bottles in a closet. When mixed, they must be stored in dark glass bottles.

When mixing them with essential oils, make small amounts only. It is a good idea to add vitamin E in the form of wheat-germ oil, in order to delay oxidation. Add 5% of the total amount.

Essential oils - the list

Angelica

Angelica is a powerful disinfectant, and speeds up the healing of cuts and sores. In addition, it has viricidal, calming, and warming properties.

It is used for treating respiratory tract problems such as colds and flu, for healing cuts and sores, and for muscle pains and arthritis.

Warning: The body must not be exposed to sunlight within 12 hours of treatment with angelica. It must not be used during pregnancy.

Anise

Trans-anethole, which is the main component of anise, has an influence on the body that resembles that of estrogen.

Anise is used mainly for treating amenorrhea (absence of menstrual periods) or PMS, as a result of its similarity to estrogen.

It blends well with coriander, lemon, and peppermint.

Warning: Anise oil has a high level of toxicity. It must not be used during pregnancy. Only people who have a great deal of knowledge of and experience in aromatherapy should use it.

Basil

Basil has disinfectant, energizing, and warming properties. It accelerates the healing of wounds.

It is used for treating respiratory tract problems such as colds, flu, and bronchitis, headaches, stings, and muscle pains.

Basil blends well with bergamot and other citrus oils, frankincense, and geranium.

Warning: Basil must not be used during pregnancy.

Benzoin

Benzoin has relaxing, warming, and expectorant properties. In addition, it speeds up the recovery of skin problems.

It is used for treating arthritis, tension and anxiety, and skin problems such as cracked skin, dry skin, irritated skin, aging skin, dermatitis, and psoriasis.

Bergamot

Bergamot has stimulating and disinfectant properties.

It is used for treating greasy skin, sores and bruises, oral herpes, psoriasis, eczema, and acne.

It blends well with most essential oils, especially with geranium, coriander, lavender, vetiver, and ylang-ylang.

Warning: It is *absolutely imperative* that the body not be exposed to sunlight within 12 hours of treatment with bergamot. Bergapten, which is one of the components of bergamot, is phototoxic, that is, it becomes toxic when exposed to the sun, and is liable to cause pigmentation spots.

However, bergapten-free bergamot oil is available, and it is safer for use. There is no need to wait before exposure to the sun after applying it.

Birch

Birch has anti-inflammatory, antiseptic, diuretic, fungicidal, and anesthetic properties.

It is used for treating muscle pains and arthritis.

Warning: Birch oil has a high level of toxicity. Only people who have a great deal of knowledge of and experience in aromatherapy should use it.

Black Pepper

Black pepper has anesthetic, antispasmodic, stimulating, and warming properties.

It is used for treating muscle pains and spasms, arthritis, and cellulite.

Black pepper blends well with frankincense, sandalwood, ginger, rose, vetiver, and citrus oils.

Warning: Black pepper must not be used during pregnancy. Because of its pungency, it should not be used on the face.

Cajeput

Cajeput has fungicidal, viricidal, antispasmodic, stimulating, and warming properties. In addition, it is a powerful disinfectant.

It is used for treating respiratory tract problems such as colds, bronchitis, sinusitis, and asthma, as well as acne, psoriasis, sores, arthritis, and stings.

Cajeput blends well with juniper, hyssop, patchouli, and vetiver.

Camphor

Camphor has stimulating and antispasmodic properties. In addition, it is a powerful antiseptic.

It is used for treating muscle pains, arthritis, acne, greasy skin, burns, sores, and bruises.

Camphor blends well with frankincense, cedarwood, cypress, and clary sage.

Warning: Camphor oil has a high level of toxicity. Asthma sufferers and pregnant women are *forbidden* to use it. Do not perform a general body massage with this oil.

The author's personal recommendation is not to use this oil at all.

Caraway

Caraway has antiseptic, antispasmodic, stimulating, and warming properties.

It is used for treating muscle pains, arthritis, greasy skin, and acne.

Caraway blends well with peppermint, fennel, cinnamon, cardamom, and ginger.

Warning: Caraway may cause irritation in sensitive skin. It must not be used during pregnancy.

Cardamom

Cardamom has stimulating, antispasmodic, diuretic, warming, and aphrodisiac properties.

It is used for treating muscle pains, fatigue, water retention, headaches, frigidity, and digestive problems such as flatulence and diarrhea.

Cardamom blends well with geranium, frankincense, juniper, myrtle, and citrus oils.

Warning: Cardamom oil may irritate sensitive skin.

Carrot Seed

Carrot seed speeds up the healing of sores and burns, and enhances sun-tanning.

It is used for treating burns, wrinkles, and aging skin.

Comment: From carrot seed, only essential oil is produced. In recent years, various weird and wonderful "carrot oils" have become common. In general, they are produced by means of the following process: Carrot powder (dried, ground carrot) is added to distilled sesame oil, which combines with the oil-soluble components in the powder (beta carotene, for example - this is the substance that gives carrot its orange color). Afterward, the powder residue is removed by straining. This is not to say that the oil is ineffective, but the name "carrot oil" in this case is pretentious and misleading.

Cedarwood

Cedarwood has antiseptic, fungicidal, stimulant, and expectorant properties.

It is used for treating hair problems such as dandruff, hair loss, and scalp diseases, as well as greasy skin, acne, eczema, tension, and anxiety.

Cedarwood blends well with bergamot, clary sage, cypress, juniper, neroli, rose, rosemary, and ylang-ylang.

Celery

Celery has stimulating, diuretic, aphrodisiac, anti-inflammatory, and anesthetic properties.

It is used for treating fatigue, arthritis, inflamed skin, and cellulite.

Celery blends well with angelica, palmarosa, basil, and citrus oils.

Chamomile

Chamomile has anesthetic, antispasmodic, anti-inflammatory, antispastic, and relaxing properties.

It is used for treating tension, anxiety, and depression, fatigue, headaches, migraines, sinusitis, scaly skin, muscle pains, arthritis, acne, irritated skin, burns, cracked, chapped skin, dermatitis, dry skin, oral herpes, inflamed skin, psoriasis, stretch marks, menstrual cramps, sores, and cuts.

Chamomile blends well with citrus oils, geranium, rose, patchouli, and ylang-ylang.

Cinnamon

Cinnamon has stimulating and antispasmodic properties. In addition, it is a powerful disinfectant.

It is used for treating respiratory tract problems such as flu and asthma, muscle pains, arthritis, stings, and lice.

It blends well with citrus oils, anise, caraway, clove, and rose.

Warning: Cinnamon oil has a high level of toxicity. It must not be used during pregnancy. As it is liable to burn, it should not be used on the face.

Citronella

Citronella is a stimulating oil that is a powerful disinfectant, and an insect repellent.

It is used for treating muscle pains, arthritis, and stings.

It blends well with citrus oils, myrtle, rosemary, and peppermint.

Clary Sage

Clary sage has anti-inflammatory, antispasmodic, viricidal, relaxing, warming, and aphrodisiac properties.

It is used for treating weakness and depression, muscle pains, menstrual cramps, bronchitis, aging skin, dermatitis, oral herpes, cuts, and burns.

Clary sage blends well with citrus oils, jasmine, cedarwood, sandalwood, vetiver, and neroli.

Warning: Clary sage must not be used during pregnancy. Do not use clary sage for several hours after the consumption of alcohol.

Comment: In spite of the above warnings, clary sage is far safer to use than regular sage *(Salvia officinalis)*.

Clove

Clove has antispasmodic, viricidal, stimulating, and warming properties. In addition, it is a powerful antiseptic.

It is used for treating toothache, gum infections, muscle pains, respiratory tract problems such as asthma and bronchitis, as well as lice, sores, and bruises.

Clove blends well with citrus oils, cinnamon, sage, and nutmeg.

Warning: Clove must not be used with babies or young children, or during pregnancy. It should always be used in small doses, as it is liable to cause skin irritations.

Coriander

Coriander has warming, stimulating, and antispasmodic properties.

It is used for treating arthritis and muscle pains.

Coriander blends well with citrus oils, marjoram, cypress, and ginger.

Warning: When coriander oil is used on the face, it must be used in minute quantities, as it is liable to irritate the skin.

Cypress

Cypress has antiseptic, contracting, and expectorant properties.

It is used for acne, greasy skin, bruises, cellulite, arthritis, and varicose veins.

Cypress blends well with juniper, lavender, pine, sandalwood, and myrrh.

Dill

Dill has disinfectant, antispasmodic, and relaxing properties. In addition, it relieves flatulence.

It is used for treating depression, sores, digestive problems such as constipation and flatulence, and respiratory tract problems such as colds and bronchitis.

Dill blends well with citrus oils, geranium, myrtle, and neroli.

Warning: Dill must not be used during pregnancy. It must not be used with babies or young children.

Eucalyptus

Eucalyptus has energizing, viricidal, stimulating, anesthetizing, and expectorant properties.

It is used for treating respiratory tract problems, acne, herpes, sores and bruises, burns, stings, and lice.

Eucalyptus blends well with pine, lavender, peppermint and lemon.

Warning: Do not use eucalyptus oil with infants or young children. (Myrtle oil, which has similar properties, but is milder, can be used with them.)

Fennel

Fennel has antispasmodic, warming, and diuretic properties. In addition, it increases cardiac capacity.

It is used for treating fatigue, gum infections, inflamed joints, muscle pains, animal bites, stings, cellulite, greasy skin, aging skin, shortage of milk during nursing, irregular menstrual periods, digestive problems such as stomach-aches and flatulence, and respiratory tract problems such as bronchitis, runny nose, and flu .

Fennel blends well with geranium, rose, cedarwood, and frankincense.

Warning: Fennel must not be used by pregnant women, people who suffer from epilepsy, or babies and young children.

Frankincense (Olibanum)

Frankincense has relaxing, stimulating, and warming properties.

It is used for treating respiratory tract problems such as colds and bronchitis, fatigue, irritated skin, aging skin, stretch marks, sores, bruises, and acne.

Frankincense blends well with most essential oils, especially sandalwood, basil, geranium, and myrrh.

Galbanum

Galbanum has stimulating, anesthetic, antispasmodic, antiflatulent, expectorant, and diuretic properties.

It is used for treating mental stress and tension, respiratory tract problems such as bronchitis and colds, muscle pains, arthritis, inflamed skin, sores, and cuts.

Galbanum blends well with lemon grass, myrrh, palmarosa, ginger, and rose.

Warning: Galbanum must not be used during pregnancy. Furthermore, it is liable to irritate sensitive skin.

Garlic

Garlic has antispasmodic, fungicidal, and viricidal properties. In addition, it is a powerful antiseptic, and destroys parasites and worms in the digestive tract.

It is used for treating muscle spasms, arthritis, respiratory tract problems such as bronchitis and colds, as well as acne, stings, and sores.

Because of its exceptionally strong odor, garlic oil is problematic as far as blending with other oils is concerned.

Warning: Garlic oil must not be used by nursing mothers. Care must be taken when it is applied to the face, as it is very pungent, and is liable to burn.

Geranium

Geranium has disinfectant properties. In addition, it speeds up the dissolving of cellulite, and combats water retention.

It is used for treating sores, burns, sunburn, and arthritis. It is also used in skin conditions such as cracked skin, dermatitis, oral herpes, acne, greasy skin, and dry, sensitive skin.

Geranium blends well with most essential oils, especially with citrus and rose oils.

Ginger

Ginger has warming and stimulating properties. It is also considered to be an aphrodisiac.

It is used for treating respiratory tract infections, arthritis, and muscle pains.

Ginger blends well with myrtle, coriander, patchouli, and vetiver.

Warning: In order to avoid skin inflammations, ginger should be used at a low concentration. It must not be used with infants or small children.

Grapefruit

Grapefruit has stimulating properties; it assists in dissolving cellulite, and eliminating liquids.

It is used for treating accumulated liquids and swelling, cellulite, greasy skin, and acne.

Grapefruit blends well with other citrus oils, geranium, cedarwood, lavender and coriander.

Warning: The body must not be exposed to sunlight within 12 hours of treatment with grapefruit.

Hyssop

Hyssop has antiseptic, antispasmodic and stimulating properties.

It is used for treating respiratory tract problems such as colds and bronchitis, sores and bruises, and dermatitis.

It blends well with citrus oils, lavender, and clary sage.

Warning: Hyssop oil has a high level of toxicity. Pregnant women, children, and people who suffer from epilepsy, or have a high fever, are *forbidden* to use it. Only people who have a great deal of knowledge of and experience in aromatherapy should use it.

Immortelle (Everlasting)

Immortelle has antispasmodic, stimulating, antiseptic, fungicidal, and expectorant properties.

It is used for treating respiratory tract problems such as bronchitis, colds, and sinusitis, as well as skin conditions such as dermatitis, psoriasis, acne, and inflamed skin.

Immortelle blends well with patchouli, yarrow, vetiver, cedarwood, cypress, clary sage, and citrus oils.

Jasmine

Jasmine is considered to be the most effective aphrodisiac of all the essential oils. It has, in addition, antispasmodic, relaxing, and warming properties, and it speeds up the regeneration of the epidermal (skin) cells.

It is used for treating frigidity, anxiety, depression, muscle pains, respiratory tract problems such as colds and asthma, as well as skin conditions, including dry, sensitive skin, irritated skin, dermatitis, and wrinkles.

Jasmine blends well with most essential oils, especially citrus oils, rose, sandalwood, palmarosa, and geranium.

Juniper

Juniper has antiseptic, antibacterial, warming, and stimulating properties. It also releases accumulated liquids.

It is used for treating muscle pains, arthritis, greasy skin, acne, dermatitis, and psoriasis.

Juniper blends well with citrus oils, geranium, lavender, myrrh, and sandalwood.

Warning: Juniper must not be used during pregnancy.

Laurel (Bay)

Laurel has relaxing, warming, disinfectant, anesthetic, and antispasmodic properties.

It is used for treating respiratory tract problems such as bronchitis and colds, as well as arthritis, muscle pains, scaly skin, and inflamed skin.

Laurel blends well with coriander, ginger, marjoram, cedarwood, rose, and lavender.

Warning: Laurel must not be used during pregnancy.

Lavender

Lavender has antiseptic, relaxing, anesthetic, and antispasmodic properties.

It is used for treating sinusitis, migraine, muscle pains, respiratory tract problems such as asthma and bronchitis, as well as skin problems including aging skin, greasy skin, hypersensitive skin, acne, dermatitis, psoriasis, burns, sores, and stings.

Lavender blends well with most essential oils, especially chamomile, frankincense, and citrus oils.

Comment: There is a range of different-quality lavender oil available. Sometimes *lavendine* oil (a hybrid of *Lavandula vera* and *Lavandula spica*) is sold as lavender oil. *Lavendine* contains five times more essential oil than lavender, but the quality is lower. For this reason, it is important to purchase lavender oil from a reliable source.

Lemon

Lemon is a powerful antiseptic, and has viricidal, fungicidal, and stimulating properties.

It is used for treating respiratory tract problems (bronchitis, colds), arthritis, cellulite, oral herpes, acne, greasy skin, psoriasis, scaly skin, and stings.

Lemon combines well with most essential oils, especially geranium, chamomile, and neroli.

Warning: The body must not be exposed to sunlight within 12 hours of treatment with lemon.

Lemon Grass

Lemon grass has relaxing, disinfectant, bactericidal, and diuretic properties. In addition, it is an effective insect repellent, and stimulates the digestive system.

It is used for treating headaches, inflamed skin, greasy skin, acne, and problems of the digestive system such as flatulence and constipation.

It blends well with citrus oils, geranium, jasmine, and lavender.

Warning: Lemon grass must not be used with babies and young children.

Comment: There is a strain of lemon grass that is called *Cymbopogon flexuosus* from which the essential oil Indian verbena is produced - quite distinct from real lemon verbena, which is incomparably more expensive.

Lemon Verbena

Lemon verbena has fungicidal, antispasmodic, relaxing and refreshing properties. It is a powerful antiseptic.

It is used for treating depression, tension, acne, and stomach-aches resulting from flatulence.

Lemon verbena blends well with citrus oils, palmarosa, jasmine, and basil.

Warning: The body must not be exposed to sunlight within 12 hours of treatment with lemon verbena. It is liable to irritate the skin.

Comment: The global production of lemon verbena is extremely limited, and for this reason it is quite expensive. It is important to purchase it from a reliable source. Ensure that the oil is indeed lemon verbena oil, and not Indian verbena (which in fact is a strain of lemon grass called *Cymbopogon flexuosus*), or Spanish verbena. There are synthetic imitations of lemon verbena oil available as well.

Lime

Lime has antiseptic, viricidal, fungicidal, and contracting properties.

It is used to treat depression and anxiety, respiratory tract problems such as colds and sinusitis, as well as muscle pains, arthritis, greasy skin, sores, and cuts.

Lime blend well with other citrus oils, lavender, palmarosa, and angelica.

Warning: The body must not be exposed to sunlight within 12 hours of treatment with lime.

Mandarin

Mandarin has viricidal and stimulating properties.

It is used for treating muscle pains, greasy skin, cellulite, and stretch marks.

Mandarin blends well with other citrus oils, geranium, cedarwood, and lavender.

Warning: The body must not be exposed to sunlight within 12 hours of treatment with mandarin.

Marigold (Tagetes)

Marigold has relaxing, stimulating, antispasmodic, fungicidal, and bactericidal properties.

It is used for treating hypersensitive skin, acne scars, burns, cuts, dermatitis, impetigo.

Marjoram

Marjoram has warming, antispasmodic, and relaxing properties. Furthermore, it is a libido suppressant.

It is used for tension and anxiety, migraines, arthritis, headaches, menstrual cramps, and respiratory tract problems such as bronchitis and colds.

Marjoram blends well with bergamot, chamomile, lavender, and coriander.

Warning: Marjoram oil must not be used during pregnancy.

Melissa

Melissa has relaxing, cooling, viricidal properties. In addition, it prevents cramps.

It is used for treating insomnia, migraines, depression, muscle pains, respiratory tract problems such as bronchitis and colds, dermatitis, stings, and sensitive, irritated skin.

Melissa blends well with myrtle, geranium, lavender, and citrus oils.

Warning: Melissa oil must not be used during pregnancy.

Comment: In order to produce one kilogram of melissa oil, several tons of the plant are required. As a result, the price of authentic melissa oil is extremely high. The oil is only produced in commercial quantities in France (a few dozen kilograms a year). Most of the oils that are sold globally under the name "melissa" are in fact a mixture of citrus oils that may (or may not) contain a minuscule amount of true melissa oil. Lemon grass oil or citronella oil that is distilled with melissa leaves is also liable to be sold under the name "melissa."

Myrrh

Myrrh has warming, relaxing, disinfectant, and antifungal properties.

It is used for treating respiratory tract problems such as bronchitis and colds, inflammations of the gums, cuts, and skin conditions such as irritated skin, acne, dermatitis, dry skin, aging skin, and wrinkles.

Myrrh blends well with cedarwood, frankincense, patchouli, neroli, sandalwood, vetiver, and rose.

Warning: Myrrh oil must not be used during pregnancy.

Myrtle

Myrtle has antiseptic, *contracting,* and expectorant properties. It is used for treating respiratory tract problems such as colds, flu, and bronchitis; it is especially recommended for children, since it is relatively mild. Myrtle is also used for treating acne and greasy skin.

Myrtle blends well with lemon, pine, lavender, and peppermint.

Neroli

Neroli has antispasmodic, viricidal, relaxing, aphrodisiac properties. In addition, it accelerates the regeneration of epidermal (skin) cells.

It is used for treating anxiety and depression, frigidity, muscle pains, and skin conditions including acne, hypersensitive skin, irritated skin, dry skin, dermatitis, and aging skin.

Neroli blends well with most essential oils, especially geranium, benzoin, chamomile, frankincense, rose, sandalwood, vetiver, and cedarwood.

Comment: One thousand kilograms of flowers are required for the production of one kilogram of neroli oil, which means that it is very expensive. Authentic neroli oil is not very common, and it is difficult to obtain. Most of the oils that are sold under the name of "neroli" are in fact petitgrain oil that may (or may not) be mixed with a minuscule amount of neroli oil.

Niaouli

Niaouli has anesthetic, fungicidal, viricidal, and stimulating properties. It is also a powerful disinfectant.

It is used for treating respiratory tract problems such as sinusitis, runny nose, colds, and bronchitis, as well as arthritis, acne, burns, stings, dermatitis, and sores.

Niaouli blends well with patchouli, myrtle, lavender and camphor.

Nutmeg

Nutmeg has antiseptic, antispasmodic, stimulating, anesthetic, and aphrodisiac properties.

It is used for treating problems of the digestive system such as flatulence and diarrhea, halitosis (bad breath), menstrual cramps, muscle pains, and arthritis.

Nutmeg blends well with cinnamon, galbanum (resin), citrus oils, and cloves.

Warning: Nutmeg must not be used during pregnancy. It may cause a burning sensation on sensitive skin. It should not be used over a prolonged period of time.

Orange

Orange has antispasmodic, viricidal, calming, and warming properties.

It is used for treating tension, depression, respiratory tract problems such as bronchitis and colds, muscle pains, dry, sensitive skin, acne, aging skin, stretch marks, and dermatitis.

Orange blends well with most essential oils, especially clary sage, coriander, geranium, rose, and vetiver.

Warning: The body must not be exposed to sunlight within 12 hours of treatment with orange.

Oregano

Oregano has relaxing, disinfectant, and analgesic properties. In addition, it accelerates the dissolving of cellulite, and repels lice.

It is used for treating muscle pains, arthritis, respiratory tract problems, cellulite, and lice.

Oregano blends well with bergamot, black pepper, and juniper.

Palmarosa

Palmarosa has antiseptic, fungicidal, and viricidal properties. In addition, it speeds up the regeneration of the epidermal (skin) cells.

It is used for treating acne (and the scars that are left by acne), wrinkles, aging skin, dry, sensitive skin, sores, and bruises.

It blends well with citrus oils, geranium, jasmine, sandalwood, and cedarwood.

Parsley

Parsley has antiseptic, antispasmodic, diuretic, expectorant, and relaxing properties. In addition, it relieves flatulence, and combats water retention.

It is used for treating cellulite, swelling, arthritis, muscle pains, digestive problems (gas), sores, bruises, and spiderweb capillaries.

Parsley blends well with citrus oils, rosemary, lavender, and marjoram.

Warning: Parsley must not be used during pregnancy. It should always be used in small doses.

Patchouli

Patchouli has antibiotic, antifungal, aphrodisiac properties. In addition, it stimulates the regeneration of epidermal (skin) cells.

It is used for treating tension and anxiety, acne, cracked skin, aging skin, dermatitis, scaly skin, greasy skin, wrinkles, oral herpes, impetigo, seborrhea, hair loss, and stretch marks.

Patchouli blends well with citrus oils, ginger, lavender, myrrh, neroli, and rose.

Peppermint

Peppermint has antispasmodic, fungicidal, viricidal, cooling, and stimulating properties. It is also a powerful antiseptic.

It is used for treating muscle pains, headaches, lice, respiratory tract problems such as asthma, bronchitis, and colds, and skin conditions including acne, dermatitis, inflamed skin, and irritated skin.

Peppermint blends well with benzoin, rosemary, basil, and eucalyptus.

Warning: Do not massage peppermint oil into the entire body at once, since this causes a sensation of extreme coldness. For the same reason, peppermint oil should not be used in the bath on its own. It should be blended with other oils.

The oil must not be used at night, as it is a stimulant, and is liable to prevent you from falling asleep. Peppermint oil must not be used during pregnancy, nor must it be used with infants and young children.

Petitgrain

Petitgrain has viricidal, relaxing, and antispasmodic properties.

It is used for treating tension and anxiety, muscle pains, acne, and greasy skin.

Petitgrain blends well with most essential oils, especially geranium, ylang-ylang, rosemary, and vetiver.

Comment: Authentic petitgrain oil is produced from the leaves of the bitter orange tree *(Citrus aurantium amara)*. It can also be produced from the leaves of other citrus fruits such as lemon, mandarin, and so on. In addition, it can be produced from the branches and unripe fruit. The finest oil comes from southern France, where it is produced from the leaves only.

Pine

Pine has strong antiseptic properties. Furthermore, it is an expectorant.

It is used for treating respiratory tract problems, arthritis, muscle pains, and fatigue.

Pine blends well with bergamot and the other citrus oils, cedarwood, cypress, geranium, lavender, and patchouli.

Red Thyme

Red thyme has stimulating, antibiotic, and anesthetic properties. In addition, it is an extremely powerful disinfectant.

It is used for treating arthritis, cellulite, infected sores, and lice.

Red thyme blends well with lavender, rosemary, geranium, and cedarwood.

Warning: When using the red strain of thyme, you must be *doubly cautious,* and use an extremely small dose in order to avoid irritating the skin. Red thyme must not be used by pregnant women, people who suffer from high blood pressure, or babies and young children.

Rose

Rose has relaxing, disinfectant, antibacterial, and aphrodisiac properties.

It is used for treating anxiety, depression, fatigue, frigidity, as well as skin conditions such as aging skin, dry, sensitive skin, dermatitis, irritated skin, and wrinkles.

Rose blends well with most other essential oils, especially chamomile, frankincense, sandalwood, patchouli, vetiver, and jasmine.

Rosemary

Rosemary has stimulating, anesthetic, viricidal, and warming properties. In addition, it is a powerful antiseptic, and a louse repellent.

It is used for treating fatigue (it is effective in improving concentration while studying for exams, etc.), scaly skin, lice, headaches, migraines, sinusitis, muscle pains, greasy skin, sores, and respiratory tract problems such as asthma, bronchitis, and flu.

Rosemary blends well with citrus oils, basil, lavender, and frankincense.

Warning: Rosemary should not be used by pregnant women, by people with high blood pressure, or by people who suffer from epilepsy.

Rosewood (Bois de Rose)

Rosewood has antiseptic, anesthetic, stimulating, and fungicidal properties.

It is used for treating sensitive skin, aging skin, and headaches.

Comment: Rosewood trees are an endangered species because of the unlimited destruction of the Brazilian rainforests. The price of the oil is increasing, and, in parallel, so are the quantities of synthetic rosewood oil that are available. For this reason, you are well advised not to use this oil at all.

Sage

Sage has stimulating, anesthetic, warming, and antispasmodic properties. It is also a powerful antiseptic.

It is used for treating weakness, muscle pains, bronchitis, dermatitis, hair loss, sores, and bruises.

Sage blends well with citrus oils, rosemary, and lavender.

Warning: Sage oil must not be used by pregnant women, epilepsy sufferers, infants or young children.

Sandalwood

Sandalwood has relaxing, aphrodisiac, anti-spasmodic, antiseptic, and expectorant properties.

It is used for treating tension and depression, bronchitis, and flu, as well as skin conditions such as acne, cracked skin, dry skin, aging skin, dermatitis, wrinkles, sun-burn, and scaly skin.

Sandalwood blends well with most essential oils, especially patchouli, myrrh, frankincense, rose, and ylang-ylang.

Comment: Sandalwood oil is produced from mature trees (30-50 years old), but because of the growing demand for this oil over the last years (particularly by perfume manufacturers), there has been an ongoing decimation of the sandalwood forests in India. The price of the oil keeps rising, and young trees are being cut down in order to produce the oil.

Siberian Fir

Siberian fir has antiseptic, relaxing, and expectorant properties.

It is used for treating respiratory tract problems such as bronchitis, colds, asthma, shortness of breath, as well as muscle pains and arthritis.

Siberian fir blends well with myrrh, rosemary, myrtle, eucalyptus, and cinnamon.

Spearmint

Spearmint has disinfectant, anti-inflammatory, and stimulating properties.

It is used for treating respiratory tract problems such as colds and bronchitis, as well as acne and inflamed skin.

Spearmint blends well with myrtle, eucalyptus, rosemary, and lavender.

Warning: Spearmint must not be used during pregnancy.

Sweet Thyme

Sweet thyme has antibiotic, disinfectant, and antispasmodic properties.

It is used for treating tension, anxiety, and fatigue, headaches, migraines, respiratory tract problems such as colds, bronchitis, sinusitis, and asthma, arthritis, dermatitis, burns, acne, and irritated, inflamed skin.

Sweet thyme blends well with citrus oils, rosemary, and myrtle.

Warning: Sweet thyme must not be used during pregnancy.

Comment: Sweet thyme is the safest oil of the thyme family.

Tangerine

Tangerine has relaxing and antispasmodic properties.

It is used for treating arthritis, muscle pains, cellulite, acne, aging skin, greasy skin, and stretch marks.

Tangerine blends well with other citrus oils, ginger, geranium, and patchouli.

Tea Tree

Tea tree has antibiotic, viricidal, and fungicidal properties. It is also an extremely efficient disinfectant.

It is used for respiratory tract problems such as bronchitis, flu, and colds, acne, oral herpes, stings, lice, scars, stretch marks, sun-burn, sores, and cuts.

Tea tree blends well with myrrh, chamomile, pine, eucalyptus, and lemon.

Vetiver

Vetiver has relaxing properties, and is also considered to be an aphrodisiac.

It is used for treating muscle pains, aging skin, acne, and greasy skin.

Vetiver blends well with myrtle, clary sage, frankincense, myrrh, ginger, and rose.

Wintergreen

Wintergreen has antiseptic, stimulating, and diuretic properties.

It is used for treating arthritis, muscle pains, and cellulite.

Warning: Wintergreen oil has a high level of toxicity. Only people who have a great deal of knowledge of and experience in aromatherapy should use it.

Yarrow

Yarrow has anti-inflammatory, antispasmodic, stimulating properties. It speeds up the healing of sores.

It is used for treating sores and cuts, irritated skin, acne, cellulite, spiderweb capillaries, and dermatitis.

Yarrow blends well with myrtle, hyssop, clary sage, and eucalyptus.

Warning: The body must not be exposed to sunlight within 12 hours of treatment with yarrow.

Ylang-ylang

Ylang-ylang has antiseptic, relaxing, and aphrodisiac properties.

It is used for treating greasy skin, mixed skin, and aging skin, and for frigidity.

Ylang-ylang blends well with cedar, patchouli, chamomile, rose, jasmine, and sandalwood.

Astrolog Publishing House

P. O. Box 1123, Hod Hasharon 45111, Israel

Tel: 972-9-7412044

Fax: 972-9-7442714

E-Mail: info@astrolog.co.il

Astrolog Web Site: www.astrolog.co.il

ISBN 965-494-104-X

Published by Astrolog Publishing House 2000

Printed in Israel

2 4 6 8 10 9 7 5 3 1